RENAL REVIVAL:

APPETIZING

RECIPES FOR

KIDNEY HEALTH

BY

DR. HENRY

JAMESON

DR. Henry Jameson

2370 Layman Court, DALLAS

GA 30132

This Book is Dedicated to my Family, and to everyone who supported me in this journey.

Table Of Content

Chapter 1: Understanding Kidney Disease and Nutrition

The Basics of Kidney Function and the Role of Nutrition in Kidney Health

The kidneys are vital organs responsible for filtering waste products and excess fluids from the blood, which are then excreted as urine. In addition to waste removal, the kidneys play a crucial role in regulating electrolyte balance, blood pressure, and the production of red blood cells.

Kidney Function:
- The nephrons, tiny filtering units within the kidneys, are responsible for filtering blood and removing waste products.
- The filtered waste and excess fluids form urine, which is then transported to the bladder for excretion.

The Role of Nutrition in Kidney Health:
- Nutrition plays a critical role in supporting kidney function and managing kidney disease.
- A balanced diet helps reduce the workload on the kidneys, minimizes the accumulation of waste products, and maintains overall health.

Key Nutrients and Kidney Health:
- Protein: While essential for overall health, excessive protein intake can strain the kidneys. Managing protein intake is crucial, especially in later stages of kidney disease.
- Sodium: Excessive sodium can lead to fluid retention and high blood pressure, both of which can strain the

kidneys. Controlling sodium intake is important for managing kidney disease.

- Potassium: Proper potassium balance is essential for heart and muscle function. However, high potassium levels can be dangerous for those with kidney disease.

- Phosphorus: Kidneys regulate phosphorus levels in the blood. In kidney disease, phosphorus levels can rise, leading to bone and heart problems.

- Fluids: Proper fluid intake is crucial for kidney function. In kidney disease, fluid intake may need to be restricted to avoid fluid overload.

Overview of Different Stages of Kidney Disease and Their Dietary Implications

Kidney disease progresses through different stages, each with its own unique dietary considerations. Understanding these stages and their dietary implications is crucial for managing kidney disease effectively. Here's an overview:

1. Stage 1: Kidney Damage with Normal or High GFR (GFR > 90 mL/min)
   - In this early stage, the kidneys may have some damage, but their function is still relatively normal.
   - Dietary focus: Managing underlying conditions (e.g., diabetes, high blood pressure) to prevent further damage.
   - Nutrition goal: Emphasizing a balanced diet to support overall health and reduce the risk of progression.

2. Stage 2: Kidney Damage with Mildly Decreased GFR (GFR 60-89 mL/min)
   - Kidney function is mildly decreased, but symptoms may not yet be apparent.
   - Dietary focus: Controlling blood pressure, blood sugar, and cholesterol levels through diet.
   - Nutrition goal: Emphasizing a heart-healthy diet that is low in sodium, saturated fats, and added sugars.

3. Stage 3: Moderate Decrease in GFR (GFR 30-59 mL/min)
   - Kidney function is significantly reduced, and symptoms may start to appear.

- Dietary focus: Restricting protein, phosphorus, and potassium intake as kidney function declines.
- Nutrition goal: Working with a dietitian to create a personalized meal plan that meets nutritional needs while managing restrictions.

4. Stage 4: Severe Decrease in GFR (GFR 15-29 mL/min)

- Kidney function is severely reduced, and symptoms are often more pronounced.
- Dietary focus: Further limiting protein, phosphorus, and potassium intake to reduce strain on the kidneys.
- Nutrition goal: Following a strict meal plan tailored to individual needs, possibly with additional fluid restrictions.

5. Stage 5: Kidney Failure (GFR < 15 mL/min or on dialysis)

- Kidneys are no longer able to function effectively, requiring dialysis or a kidney transplant.
- Dietary focus: Adhering to a specialized diet to support dialysis treatment or prepare for a transplant.
- Nutrition goal: Working closely with a healthcare team to manage nutritional needs during advanced kidney disease.

Importance of a Kidney-Friendly Diet for Managing Symptoms and Slowing Disease Progression

A kidney-friendly diet plays a crucial role in managing symptoms and slowing the progression of kidney disease. Here's why it's essential:

1. Minimizing Stress on the Kidneys: A kidney-friendly diet helps reduce the workload on the kidneys by controlling the intake of certain nutrients like protein, sodium, potassium, and phosphorus. This can help slow down the decline in kidney function and manage symptoms such as fluid retention, high blood pressure, and electrolyte imbalances.

2. Managing Complications: Kidney disease can lead to various complications such as bone disease, anemia, and cardiovascular issues. A well-planned diet can help manage these complications by addressing nutritional deficiencies and promoting overall health.

3. Preventing Further Damage: Certain dietary factors can exacerbate kidney damage. For example, excessive protein intake can strain the kidneys, while high sodium levels can lead to fluid retention and elevated blood pressure. A kidney-friendly diet aims to minimize these risks and prevent further damage to the kidneys.

4. Improving Quality of Life: Following a kidney-friendly diet can improve the overall quality of life for individuals with kidney disease. By managing symptoms and slowing disease progression, it can help individuals feel better and maintain a higher level of functioning.

5. Supporting Overall Health: A kidney-friendly diet is not only beneficial for kidney health but also for overall health. It promotes a balanced intake of essential nutrients, which can benefit other organs and systems in the body.

Chapter 2: Key Nutrients for

Kidney Health

Understanding the Role of Protein, Sodium, Potassium, Phosphorus, and Fluid Intake in Kidney Disease

Proper management of key nutrients is essential in supporting kidney health and managing kidney disease. Here's a closer look at the role of each nutrient:

Balancing key nutrients is crucial for managing kidney disease and supporting overall health. Here's how to balance these nutrients in the diet:

1. Protein: Protein is an essential nutrient for the body, but it can put stress on the kidneys if consumed in excess. For individuals with kidney disease, it's important to manage protein intake to reduce strain on the kidneys. This can be achieved by focusing on high-quality protein sources such as lean meats, poultry, fish, eggs, and plant-based sources like beans and legumes. Portion control is key, and it may be necessary to work with a dietitian to determine the appropriate amount of protein for individual needs.

2. Sodium: Sodium can lead to fluid retention and high blood pressure, both of which can worsen kidney disease. Limiting sodium intake is crucial for managing these symptoms. This involves avoiding processed and packaged foods that are high in sodium, using herbs and spices to flavor food instead of salt, and being mindful of condiments and sauces that may contain hidden sodium.

3. Potassium: Potassium plays a vital role in muscle function and heart health, but too much potassium can be harmful for individuals with kidney disease, especially if their kidneys are not functioning properly. Foods high in potassium, such as bananas, oranges,

potatoes, and tomatoes, should be limited or avoided, depending on individual potassium levels. Cooking methods like leaching and soaking can help reduce potassium content in some foods.

4. Phosphorus: Phosphorus levels can rise in the blood as kidney function declines, leading to bone and heart problems. Managing phosphorus intake involves avoiding foods that are high in phosphorus, such as dairy products, nuts, seeds, and whole grains. Phosphorus additives in processed foods should also be minimized. Some individuals may require phosphorus binders to help control phosphorus levels.

5. Fluids: Fluid intake may need to be restricted for individuals with advanced kidney disease, especially if they are experiencing fluid retention or swelling. Monitoring fluid intake and being mindful of sources of hidden fluids, such as soups and fruits, can help manage fluid balance.

Recommended Daily Allowances and Guidelines for Each Nutrient

To maintain optimal kidney health, it's essential to be mindful of several key nutrients and their recommended daily allowances. Here are the recommended daily allowances and guidelines for each nutrient:

1. Protein: Protein is vital for maintaining muscle mass and overall health, but excessive protein intake can strain the kidneys. For individuals with kidney disease, the recommended daily protein intake may be lower than for the general population. Guidelines often suggest limiting protein to about 0.6 to 0.8 grams per kilogram of body weight per day, but this can vary based on individual health status and stage of kidney disease.

2. Sodium: Sodium can contribute to fluid retention and elevated blood pressure, both of which can strain the kidneys. The recommended daily sodium intake for individuals with kidney disease is often limited to

1,500 to 2,300 milligrams per day, depending on the severity of kidney impairment and other health factors.

3. Potassium: Potassium is important for nerve and muscle function, but too much potassium can be dangerous for individuals with kidney disease, especially those with impaired kidney function. Guidelines often recommend limiting potassium intake to around 2,000 to 3,000 milligrams per day, but this can vary based on individual health status and medications.

4. Phosphorus: Phosphorus is essential for bone health, but excessive phosphorus can be harmful to individuals with kidney disease, as impaired kidneys may struggle to remove it from the blood. Guidelines often suggest limiting phosphorus intake to around 800 to 1,000 milligrams per day, depending on individual health status and stage of kidney disease.

5. Fluids: Managing fluid intake is crucial for individuals with kidney disease, especially those with impaired kidney function who may have difficulty excreting excess fluids. Guidelines often recommend limiting fluid intake to around 1.5 to 2 liters per day,

but this can vary based on individual health status and stage of kidney disease.

6. Other Nutrients: Other nutrients like calcium, vitamin D, and iron also play essential roles in kidney health. Guidelines for these nutrients may vary based on individual health status and specific dietary needs.

Consulting with a healthcare professional or a registered dietitian who specializes in kidney disease can help individuals develop a personalized nutrition plan that meets their specific dietary needs and health goals.

Chapter 3: Planning a Kidney-Friendly Diet

How to Create a Personalized Meal Plan Based on Individual Needs and Dietary Restrictions

Creating a personalized meal plan for kidney health involves understanding individual dietary needs and restrictions related to kidney disease. Here are the steps to create a personalized meal plan:

1. Assessment of Dietary Needs: Begin by assessing individual dietary needs, including nutritional requirements, food preferences, and any dietary

restrictions related to kidney disease. Consider factors such as age, gender, weight, stage of kidney disease, and presence of other health conditions.

2. Consultation with a Healthcare Professional: It is important to consult with a healthcare professional, such as a registered dietitian or a healthcare provider specializing in kidney disease. They can provide personalized guidance based on individual health status and dietary requirements.

3. Understanding Nutritional Guidelines: Gain an understanding of the nutritional guidelines for kidney health, including recommendations for protein, sodium, potassium, phosphorus, fluid intake, and other nutrients. These guidelines will serve as the foundation for building a kidney-friendly meal plan.

4. Meal Planning Principles: Learn about meal planning principles for kidney health, such as portion control, balancing nutrients, and choosing foods with lower levels of phosphorus, potassium, and sodium. Emphasize whole foods and minimize processed foods in the meal plan.

5. Food Choices: Identify kidney-friendly food choices that align with individual dietary needs and preferences. This includes choosing lean protein sources, incorporating a variety of fruits and vegetables, selecting whole grains, and being mindful of portion sizes.

6. Meal Plan Development: Develop a structured meal plan that includes a variety of foods from all food groups while adhering to the recommended nutritional guidelines for kidney health. This may involve planning meals and snacks for each day of the week, considering factors such as cooking methods and food preparation.

7. Monitoring and Adjusting: Continuously monitor the effectiveness of the meal plan and make adjustments as needed based on changes in health status, dietary requirements, or individual preferences. Regular follow-ups with a healthcare professional can help ensure that the meal plan remains appropriate and effective.

8. Education and Support: Provide education and support to individuals following the meal plan, including information on food labels, cooking

techniques, and strategies for dining out. Encourage adherence to the meal plan while offering flexibility to accommodate individual needs and preferences.

Tips for Reading Food Labels to Identify Kidney-Friendly Foods

Reading food labels is essential when planning a kidney-friendly diet. Here are some tips to help you navigate food labels and identify kidney-friendly foods:

1. Check the Serving Size: Pay attention to the serving size listed on the label. The nutritional information provided is based on this serving size, so be mindful of how much you are actually consuming.

2. Review the Nutrient Content: Look for key nutrients like protein, sodium, potassium, phosphorus, and fluid content. Compare these values to your recommended daily allowances to ensure that the food aligns with your dietary goals.

3. Watch for Hidden Sodium: Sodium can be found in many processed and packaged foods. Look for terms like sodium chloride, monosodium glutamate (MSG), baking soda, and sodium nitrate on the ingredient list, as these indicate the presence of sodium.

4. Consider Phosphorus Additives: Phosphorus additives, such as phosphoric acid or sodium phosphate, can contribute to phosphorus intake. These additives are commonly found in processed foods, so check the ingredient list for them.

5. Look for Low-Potassium Options: If you need to limit potassium, look for foods labeled as low-potassium or that have a low potassium content per serving.

6. Check for Phosphorus Additives: Some food additives, such as phosphoric acid and sodium phosphate, can increase phosphorus levels in the body. Look for these additives in the ingredient list.

7. Be Mindful of Fluid Content: If you need to limit fluid intake, consider the fluid content of foods. Foods with high water content, such as soups and juicy fruits, can contribute to your daily fluid allowance.

8. Consider Overall Nutritional Value: In addition to specific nutrients, consider the overall nutritional value of the food. Choose foods that are rich in vitamins, minerals, and other essential nutrients to support overall health.

Products that often contain hidden sodium include:

1. Canned Soups: Many canned soups, especially those labeled as "ready-to-eat" or "instant," can be high in sodium to enhance flavor and preserve shelf life.

2. Processed Meats: Deli meats, sausages, bacon, and other processed meats are often cured with sodium-containing additives for flavor and preservation.

3. Canned Vegetables: Canned vegetables may be processed with added salt for preservation, so it's essential to check the label for sodium content.

4. Baked Goods: Commercially prepared baked goods like bread, muffins, and cakes may contain added sodium for flavor and texture.

5. Condiments and Sauces: Condiments like ketchup, soy sauce, barbecue sauce, and salad dressings can be high in sodium. Reduced-sodium or sodium-free versions are available as alternatives.

6. Cheese: Some types of cheese, especially processed and aged varieties, can be high in sodium.

7. Snack Foods: Potato chips, pretzels, popcorn, and other snack foods are often seasoned with salt for flavor.

8. Frozen Meals: Many frozen meals, including microwaveable dinners and entrees, are high in sodium to enhance flavor and act as a preservative.

9. Instant Noodles and Pasta: Instant noodles and pasta dishes often contain high amounts of sodium in their seasoning packets.

10. Canned Fish: Canned fish, such as tuna and salmon, may be processed with added salt for flavor and preservation.

Sample meal plans and recipes for different stages of kidney disease

7-day sample meal plan for individuals in the early stages of kidney disease (Stages 1-2).

This plan focuses on balancing nutrient intake while limiting sodium, potassium, and phosphorus:

Day 1:
- Breakfast: Scrambled eggs with spinach and mushrooms, whole-grain toast, and a small serving of mixed berries.
- Lunch: Grilled chicken salad with mixed greens, cherry tomatoes, cucumbers, and a vinaigrette dressing.

- Dinner: Baked salmon with steamed asparagus and quinoa, followed by a small serving of melon for dessert.

 Day 2:
- Breakfast: Oatmeal made with low-fat milk, topped with sliced bananas and a sprinkle of cinnamon.
- Lunch: Turkey and avocado wrap with whole-grain tortilla, served with a side of carrot sticks and hummus.
- Dinner: Baked chicken breast with roasted sweet potatoes and green beans, accompanied by a small salad.

 Day 3:
- Breakfast: Greek yogurt with honey, almonds, and a handful of blueberries.
- Lunch: Lentil soup with a side of whole-grain bread and a mixed greens salad.
- Dinner: Grilled shrimp with quinoa pilaf and steamed broccoli, followed by a small serving of applesauce for dessert.

 Day 4:
- Breakfast: Whole-grain toast with almond butter and sliced strawberries.

- Lunch: Tuna salad made with low-sodium mayonnaise, served on a bed of lettuce with a side of crackers.
- Dinner: Baked pork loin with roasted carrots and a small portion of brown rice, followed by a serving of mixed fruit for dessert.

Day 5:
- Breakfast: Smoothie made with low-potassium fruits like berries, a small amount of low-fat yogurt, and a handful of spinach.
- Lunch: Grilled vegetable and quinoa salad with a light vinaigrette dressing.
- Dinner: Baked cod with sautéed spinach and a side of couscous, followed by a small serving of sliced peaches for dessert.

Day 6:
- Breakfast: Cottage cheese with sliced peaches and a sprinkle of chopped nuts.
- Lunch: Chicken and vegetable stir-fry with a side of brown rice.
- Dinner: Beef stew with root vegetables and a slice of whole-grain bread, followed by a small serving of mixed berries for dessert.

Day 7:
- Breakfast: Whole-grain waffles with a small amount of maple syrup and a side of fresh fruit.
- Lunch: Spinach and feta cheese omelet with a side salad.
- Dinner: Grilled turkey burger with a whole-grain bun, served with a side of green beans and a small portion of potato salad made with a low-sodium dressing.

7-day meal plan for individuals with moderate-stage kidney disease (Stages 3-4).

This plan is designed to be kidney-friendly, with careful consideration of protein, sodium, potassium, and phosphorus levels:

Day 1
- Breakfast: Oatmeal made with low-fat milk, topped with sliced strawberries and a sprinkle of cinnamon.
- Lunch: Grilled chicken breast salad with mixed greens, cherry tomatoes, cucumbers, and a vinaigrette dressing.
- Dinner: Baked salmon with steamed asparagus and quinoa, followed by a small serving of melon for dessert.

Day 2
- Breakfast: Scrambled eggs with spinach and mushrooms, whole-grain toast, and a small serving of mixed berries.
- Lunch: Turkey and avocado wrap with whole-grain tortilla, served with a side of carrot sticks and hummus.
- Dinner: Baked chicken breast with roasted sweet potatoes and green beans, accompanied by a small salad.

Day 3
- Breakfast: Smoothie made with low-fat yogurt, banana, and a handful of spinach.
- Lunch: Tuna salad made with low-sodium mayonnaise, served on a bed of lettuce with a side of crackers.
- Dinner: Stir-fried tofu with mixed vegetables and brown rice, followed by a serving of baked apples for dessert.

Day 4
- Breakfast: Cottage cheese with sliced peaches and a sprinkle of cinnamon.
- Lunch: Quinoa salad with chickpeas, diced vegetables, and a lemon vinaigrette dressing.

- Dinner: Grilled shrimp skewers with grilled zucchini and a small serving of wild rice, followed by a fruit salad for dessert.

Day 5
- Breakfast: Greek yogurt with honey and mixed berries.
- Lunch: Lentil soup with a side of whole-grain bread.
- Dinner: Baked cod with steamed broccoli and a quinoa pilaf, followed by a small serving of mixed fruit for dessert.

Day 6
- Breakfast: Whole-grain toast with almond butter and sliced banana.
- Lunch: Chicken and vegetable stir-fry with brown rice.
- Dinner: Grilled pork tenderloin with roasted vegetables and a small green salad, followed by a fruit cup for dessert.

Day 7
- Breakfast: Scrambled eggs with diced tomatoes and spinach, served with a slice of whole-grain toast.
- Lunch: Greek salad with grilled chicken breast and a lemon vinaigrette dressing.

- Dinner: Baked turkey meatballs with marinara sauce, served with whole-wheat pasta and a side of steamed green beans, followed by a small serving of fruit salad for dessert.

7-day sample meal plan for someone with advanced stage kidney disease (Stage 5, Pre-Dialysis).

This meal plan is designed to be kidney-friendly, focusing on controlling protein, sodium, potassium, phosphorus, and fluid intake:

Day 1
- Breakfast:
  - Scrambled eggs made with egg whites, topped with chopped tomatoes and spinach.
  - 1 slice of whole-grain toast.
  - 1 small apple.
- Lunch:
  - Tuna salad with low-sodium mayonnaise, mixed greens, and cucumber.
  - 1 serving of unsalted crackers.
- Dinner:
  - Baked chicken breast.
  - Steamed green beans.

- 1/2 cup of cooked white rice.

- 1 small pear.

Day 2
- Breakfast:
  - Oatmeal made with water, topped with sliced bananas and a sprinkle of cinnamon.
  - 1/2 cup of low-fat milk.
- Lunch:
  - Grilled salmon.
  - Quinoa salad with diced bell peppers and a light vinaigrette dressing.
- Dinner:
  - Stir-fried tofu with mixed vegetables.
  - 1/2 cup of cooked white rice.
  - 1 small orange.

Day 3
- Breakfast:
  - Greek yogurt with a drizzle of honey.
  - 1 small apple.
- Lunch:
  - Turkey and avocado wrap with whole-grain tortilla.
  - Carrot sticks with hummus.
- Dinner:
  - Baked cod.

- Steamed asparagus.
- 1/2 cup of cooked quinoa.
- 1 small peach.

Day 4
- Breakfast:
- Smoothie made with low-potassium fruits like berries, a small amount of low-fat yogurt, and a handful of spinach.
- Lunch:
- Chicken salad with mixed greens, cherry tomatoes, and a light vinaigrette dressing.
- Dinner:
- Lentil soup.
- 1 slice of whole-grain bread.
- 1 small apple.

Day 5
- Breakfast:
- Scrambled eggs made with egg whites, topped with chopped tomatoes and spinach.
- 1 slice of whole-grain toast.
- Lunch:
- Tuna salad with low-sodium mayonnaise, mixed greens, and cucumber.
- 1 serving of unsalted crackers.

- Dinner:
  - Baked chicken breast.
  - Steamed green beans.
  - 1/2 cup of cooked white rice.
  - 1 small pear.

Day 6
- Breakfast:
  - Oatmeal made with water, topped with sliced
bananas and a sprinkle of cinnamon.
  - 1/2 cup of low-fat milk.
- Lunch:
  - Grilled salmon.
  - Quinoa salad with diced bell peppers and a light
vinaigrette dressing.
- Dinner:
  - Stir-fried tofu with mixed vegetables.
  - 1/2 cup of cooked white rice.
  - 1 small orange.

Day 7
- Breakfast:
  - Greek yogurt with a drizzle of honey.
  - 1 small apple.
- Lunch:
  - Turkey and avocado wrap with whole-grain tortilla.

- Carrot sticks with hummus.
- Dinner:
  - Baked cod.
  - Steamed asparagus.
  - 1/2 cup of cooked quinoa.
  - 1 small peach.

Remember to adjust portion sizes and food choices based on individual dietary needs and preferences. It's essential to work closely with a healthcare professional or a registered dietitian to ensure that the meal plan meets your specific nutritional needs and health goals.

7-day meal plan for patients on dialysis.

This plan is designed to be kidney-friendly, low in sodium, potassium, and phosphorus, and tailored for those with advanced kidney disease requiring dialysis. It's important to note that individual dietary needs may vary, so it's best to consult with a healthcare professional or a registered dietitian for personalized meal planning.

Day 1

- Breakfast: Scrambled eggs with low-potassium vegetables (such as bell peppers and onions), whole-grain toast, and a small serving of strawberries.
- Lunch: Grilled chicken breast salad with mixed greens, cherry tomatoes, cucumbers, and a low-sodium dressing.
- Dinner: Baked salmon with steamed green beans, brown rice, and a small side salad.

Day 2
- Breakfast: Oatmeal made with low-fat milk, topped with sliced bananas and a sprinkle of cinnamon.
- Lunch: Turkey and avocado wrap with a whole-grain tortilla, served with a side of carrot sticks and hummus.
- Dinner: Stir-fried tofu with mixed vegetables (low-potassium options like bell peppers, onions, and snap peas) and quinoa.

Day 3
- Breakfast: Greek yogurt with a small amount of honey, mixed berries, and a sprinkle of chia seeds.
- Lunch: Lentil soup with a side of whole-grain bread and a small green salad.
- Dinner: Grilled chicken breast with roasted sweet potatoes, steamed broccoli, and a side of applesauce.

Day 4

- Breakfast: Spinach and feta cheese omelet, whole-grain toast, and a small serving of melon.
- Lunch: Tuna salad made with low-sodium mayonnaise, served on a bed of lettuce with a side of crackers.
- Dinner: Baked cod with lemon and herbs, steamed asparagus, quinoa, and a small side salad.

Day 5

- Breakfast: Smoothie made with low-potassium fruits (like berries), a small amount of low-fat yogurt, and spinach.
- Lunch: Chicken and vegetable stir-fry with brown rice.
- Dinner: Baked chicken thighs with roasted Brussels sprouts, whole-grain pasta, and a small green salad.

Day 6

- Breakfast: Cottage cheese with sliced peaches and a sprinkle of chopped nuts.
- Lunch: Egg salad sandwich made with low-sodium bread and a side of carrot sticks.

- Dinner: Beef and vegetable kebabs with bell peppers, onions, and cherry tomatoes, served with a small serving of rice.

Day 7
- Breakfast: Whole-grain pancakes with a small amount of syrup and a side of fresh fruit.
- Lunch: Veggie burger on a whole-grain bun with lettuce, tomato, and a side of baked potato (with the skin removed).
- Dinner: Roasted turkey breast with mashed potatoes (made with low-potassium milk) and steamed green beans.

Chapter 4: Managing

Protein Intake

Understanding the Role of Protein

in Kidney Disease

Protein is an essential nutrient that plays a crucial role in maintaining overall health, including the health of your kidneys. However, for individuals with kidney disease, managing protein intake is critical to prevent further damage to the kidneys and to maintain overall health. Here's what you need to know about the role of protein in kidney disease:

1. Building Blocks of Life: Proteins are the building blocks of life, essential for the growth, repair, and maintenance of body tissues. They are made up of

amino acids, which are essential for various bodily functions.

2. Kidney Function: Your kidneys play a key role in filtering waste products and excess fluids from your blood, but they also help regulate the balance of certain nutrients, including protein. When your kidneys are functioning properly, they can effectively filter out waste products from protein metabolism.

3. Protein Metabolism: When you consume protein, your body breaks it down into amino acids, which are then used for various functions, such as building and repairing tissues, producing enzymes and hormones, and supporting the immune system. However, the waste products of protein metabolism, such as urea and creatinine, need to be excreted by the kidneys.

4. Impact of Kidney Disease: In individuals with kidney disease, the kidneys may not be able to effectively filter out the waste products of protein metabolism, leading to a buildup of toxins in the blood. This can put additional strain on the kidneys and contribute to further kidney damage.

5. Managing Protein Intake: Depending on the stage of kidney disease and the level of kidney function, your healthcare provider may recommend adjusting your protein intake. In some cases, a lower-protein diet may be recommended to reduce the workload on the kidneys and slow the progression of kidney disease. However, it's important to ensure that you still get enough high-quality protein to meet your nutritional needs.

6. High-Quality Protein Sources: When managing protein intake in kidney disease, it's important to focus on high-quality protein sources that are easier on the kidneys. These include lean meats, poultry, fish, eggs, dairy products, and plant-based sources of protein like beans, lentils, and tofu.

Strategies for Managing Protein Intake While Maintaining Nutritional Needs

Protein is an essential nutrient for maintaining muscle mass, supporting immune function, and repairing tissues. However, for individuals with kidney disease, especially those on dialysis, managing protein intake is crucial to prevent the build-up of waste products in the blood. Here are some strategies for managing protein intake while maintaining nutritional needs:

1. Choose High-Quality Protein Sources: Opt for high-quality protein sources that are lower in phosphorus and potassium. Examples include lean meats (like chicken, turkey, and fish), eggs, dairy products (such as milk, yogurt, and cheese), and plant-based proteins like tofu and legumes.

2. Monitor Portion Sizes: Pay attention to portion sizes to ensure you're getting enough protein without consuming excessive amounts. A healthcare

professional or dietitian can help determine the appropriate amount of protein for your individual needs.

3. Balance Protein Intake Throughout the Day: Instead of consuming a large amount of protein in one meal, spread your protein intake throughout the day. This can help optimize protein utilization and reduce the workload on the kidneys.

4. Limit Phosphorus-Rich Proteins: Some high-protein foods are also rich in phosphorus, which can be problematic for individuals with kidney disease. Limiting phosphorus-rich proteins like dairy products, nuts, and seeds can help manage phosphorus levels in the blood.

5. Consider Protein Supplements: In some cases, protein supplements may be necessary to meet protein needs without consuming excessive phosphorus and potassium. However, it's essential to choose supplements that are specifically designed for individuals with kidney disease and to use them under the guidance of a healthcare professional.

6. Monitor Kidney Function: Regular monitoring of kidney function is essential for individuals with kidney disease, especially those on dialysis. Changes in kidney function may necessitate adjustments to protein intake to ensure that nutritional needs are being met without putting undue stress on the kidneys.

7. Work with a Dietitian: A registered dietitian who specializes in kidney disease can help you develop a personalized meal plan that meets your nutritional needs while managing protein intake. They can also provide guidance on food choices, portion sizes, and meal planning to support kidney health.

High-Quality Protein Sources and Portion Control Recommendations

Protein is an essential nutrient for overall health, but for individuals with kidney disease, managing protein intake is crucial to reduce the strain on the kidneys. Here are some high-quality protein sources and portion control recommendations to help manage protein intake:

High-Quality Protein Sources:

1. Egg Whites: Egg whites are an excellent source of high-quality protein and are lower in phosphorus compared to whole eggs. They can be used in various dishes like omelets, scrambles, and baked goods.

2. Skinless Poultry: Chicken and turkey without the skin are lean sources of protein. They can be grilled, baked, or roasted for a healthy meal option.

3. Fish: Fish like salmon, trout, and tuna are rich in omega-3 fatty acids and high-quality protein. They can be baked or grilled for a delicious and nutritious meal.

4. Dairy Products: Low-fat or fat-free dairy products like milk, yogurt, and cheese can be good sources of protein. However, it's important to choose lower phosphorus options and limit intake based on individual needs.

5. Lean Meats: Lean cuts of beef and pork can provide high-quality protein. Trimming visible fat and choosing lean cuts can help reduce saturated fat intake.

6. Plant-Based Proteins: Beans, lentils, and tofu are excellent sources of plant-based protein. They are also lower in phosphorus and can be incorporated into a variety of dishes.

Portion Control Recommendations:

1. Monitor Portion Sizes: Keeping an eye on portion sizes is essential for managing protein intake. Use measuring cups or a food scale to ensure accurate portions.

2. Balance Protein Intake: Aim for a balanced intake of protein throughout the day rather than consuming large amounts in one meal. This can help reduce the workload on the kidneys.

3. Adjust Based on Kidney Function: Individuals with advanced kidney disease may need to further restrict protein intake. Work with a dietitian to determine the appropriate level of protein for your specific needs.

4. Consider Protein Supplements: In some cases, protein supplements may be recommended to meet protein needs without increasing the workload on the kidneys. However, this should be done under the guidance of a healthcare professional.

Chapter 5: Controlling Sodium Intake

The Impact of Sodium on Kidney Function and Blood Pressure

Sodium plays a crucial role in maintaining fluid balance and nerve function in the body. However, excessive sodium intake can have detrimental effects on kidney function and blood pressure, especially for individuals with kidney disease. Here's how sodium impacts kidney function and blood pressure:

1. Fluid Retention: Sodium has the ability to retain water in the body, leading to fluid retention. For individuals with impaired kidney function, the kidneys

may struggle to excrete excess sodium, resulting in fluid buildup and swelling (edema).

2. Increased Blood Pressure: High sodium intake can elevate blood pressure, which can be particularly harmful for individuals with kidney disease. Elevated blood pressure can further damage the kidneys and increase the risk of cardiovascular complications.

3. Kidney Damage: Excessive sodium intake can contribute to kidney damage over time. The kidneys play a crucial role in filtering out waste products and maintaining electrolyte balance, and high sodium levels can strain the kidneys, leading to progressive damage.

4. Risk of Heart Disease: High sodium intake is associated with an increased risk of heart disease, which is a common complication of kidney disease. Managing sodium intake is important for reducing the risk of cardiovascular complications.

Strategies for Controlling Sodium Intake:

1. Read Food Labels: Pay attention to the sodium content listed on food labels. Choose low-sodium or sodium-free options whenever possible.

2. Limit Processed Foods: Processed and packaged foods are often high in sodium. Opt for fresh, whole foods and limit the consumption of processed items like canned soups, sauces, and snacks.

3. Use Herbs and Spices: Flavor foods with herbs, spices, and other seasonings instead of relying on salt for flavor. This can add variety to meals without increasing sodium intake.

4. Cook at Home: Cooking meals at home allows you to control the amount of sodium in your food. Use less salt during cooking and at the table.

5. Rinse Canned Foods: If using canned foods, such as beans or vegetables, rinse them under running water to remove excess sodium.

6. Limit Condiments: Condiments like soy sauce, ketchup, and salad dressings can be high in sodium. Use them sparingly or look for low-sodium alternatives.

Tips for Reducing Sodium in the Diet While Maintaining Flavor

Reducing sodium intake is crucial for managing blood pressure and fluid balance, especially for individuals with kidney disease. However, cutting back on sodium doesn't mean sacrificing flavor. Here are some tips for reducing sodium in the diet while maintaining flavor:

Cooking Tips:

1. Use Herbs and Spices: Experiment with a variety of herbs and spices to add flavor to your meals without relying on salt. Popular choices include basil, oregano, garlic powder, onion powder, cumin, and turmeric.

2. Lemon or Lime Juice: Citrus juices like lemon or lime can add a refreshing zest to dishes. They can be used in marinades, dressings, or as a finishing touch to enhance flavor.

3. Vinegar: Vinegar, especially balsamic or apple cider vinegar, can add a tangy flavor to dishes. Use it in salads, sauces, or as a marinade for meats and vegetables.

4. Low-Sodium Broth or Stock: When cooking soups, stews, or sauces, opt for low-sodium or homemade broth or stock. This allows you to control the amount of salt added to your dishes.

Dining Tips:

1. Read Labels: When purchasing packaged or processed foods, read the labels carefully and choose products with lower sodium content. Look for "low-sodium" or "no added salt" options.

2. Limit Condiments: Many condiments like soy sauce, ketchup, and salad dressings are high in sodium. Use them sparingly or look for low-sodium versions.

3. Fresh Ingredients: Whenever possible, opt for fresh fruits, vegetables, and meats instead of canned or processed options. Fresh foods tend to be lower in sodium.

4. Cook at Home: Cooking meals at home allows you to control the amount of salt added to your dishes. Use salt-free seasonings and taste your food as you cook to adjust flavors.

Dining Out Tips:

1. Ask for Modifications: When dining out, don't hesitate to ask for modifications to your meal to reduce sodium. Request sauces and dressings on the side, and ask for your dish to be prepared without added salt.

2. Choose Wisely: Look for menu items that are naturally lower in sodium, such as grilled or steamed dishes. Avoid dishes that are heavily processed or fried, as they tend to be higher in sodium.

3. Be Mindful of Portions: Restaurant portions are often larger than necessary. Consider sharing a meal or packing half of it to take home to reduce sodium intake.

Chapter 6: Monitoring Potassium Levels

Understanding the Role of Potassium in Kidney Disease and Heart Health

Potassium is an essential mineral that plays a vital role in various bodily functions, including muscle contraction, nerve signaling, and fluid balance. However, for individuals with kidney disease, especially those with advanced kidney impairment, managing potassium levels is crucial due to the risk of hyperkalemia (high potassium levels), which can be harmful to the heart and other organs. Here's an overview of the role of potassium in kidney disease and heart health:

Role of Potassium in Kidney Disease:

1. Fluid Balance: Potassium helps maintain fluid balance in the body by regulating the movement of fluids in and out of cells. In individuals with impaired kidney function, the kidneys may struggle to excrete excess potassium, leading to elevated levels in the blood.

2. Muscle Function: Potassium is essential for proper muscle function, including the contraction and relaxation of muscles. Imbalances in potassium levels can lead to muscle weakness, cramping, and in severe cases, paralysis.

3. Heart Health: Potassium plays a crucial role in heart function, helping to regulate the heartbeat and maintain normal heart rhythm. Elevated potassium levels can affect the electrical signals in the heart, leading to irregular heartbeats or even cardiac arrest.

Managing Potassium Intake:

1. Dietary Sources: Potassium is found in many foods, with particularly high levels in fruits, vegetables, and legumes. While these foods are generally healthy, they can be high in potassium, making portion control important for individuals with kidney disease.

2. Monitoring Levels: Regular monitoring of potassium levels through blood tests is essential for individuals with kidney disease. This allows healthcare providers to assess potassium levels and make dietary or medication adjustments as needed.

3. Medication Management: Some medications, such as certain blood pressure medications and potassium-sparing diuretics, can affect potassium levels. It's important to discuss medication management with a healthcare provider to ensure that potassium levels are carefully monitored.

4. Symptom Awareness: Being aware of symptoms of high potassium levels, such as weakness, fatigue, irregular heartbeat, and numbness or tingling, is crucial. Promptly reporting any concerning symptoms to a healthcare provider can help prevent complications.

How to Manage Potassium Intake Through Food Choices

For individuals with kidney disease, especially those on dialysis, monitoring potassium intake is crucial to prevent hyperkalemia (high potassium levels), which can lead to serious health complications. Here are some strategies to manage potassium intake through food choices:

1. Know High-Potassium Foods: Be aware of foods that are high in potassium, such as bananas, oranges, potatoes, tomatoes, and certain dried fruits. These foods should be consumed in moderation or avoided, depending on individual potassium restrictions.

2. Choose Low-Potassium Alternatives: Opt for low-potassium alternatives to high-potassium foods. For example, choose apples or berries instead of bananas for a lower-potassium fruit option.

3. Limit Potassium-Rich Ingredients: Limit the use of potassium-rich ingredients in cooking, such as tomato

paste, tomato sauce, and certain types of salt substitutes that contain potassium chloride.

4. Use Cooking Methods to Reduce Potassium: Some cooking methods can help reduce the potassium content of foods. For example, boiling potatoes can remove some of the potassium, making them lower in potassium than when they are baked or fried.

5. Read Food Labels: Pay attention to food labels and choose products that are labeled as low-potassium or potassium-free. Food labels can provide valuable information about the potassium content of packaged foods.

6. Portion Control: Even lower-potassium foods can contribute to high potassium levels if consumed in large quantities. Practice portion control and be mindful of serving sizes to manage potassium intake.

7. Work with a Dietitian: A registered dietitian who specializes in kidney disease can help create a personalized meal plan that takes individual potassium restrictions into account. They can provide guidance on food choices and portion sizes to manage potassium intake effectively.

8. Monitor Blood Potassium Levels: Regularly monitor blood potassium levels as recommended by your healthcare provider. This can help track the effectiveness of dietary changes and ensure that potassium levels remain within a safe range.

Foods to Limit or Avoid for Those with High Potassium Levels

Potassium is a mineral that plays a vital role in muscle function and maintaining proper fluid balance in the body. However, for individuals with kidney disease, especially those with high potassium levels (hyperkalemia), it is essential to monitor and manage potassium intake. Here are some foods to limit or avoid for those with high potassium levels:

1. Bananas: Bananas are known for their high potassium content. While they are a healthy fruit choice for many people, individuals with kidney disease and high potassium levels should consume them in moderation or avoid them altogether.

2. Oranges and Orange Juice: Oranges and orange juice are rich in potassium. Instead of oranges, consider consuming lower-potassium fruits like apples, berries, or grapes.

3. Potatoes: Potatoes, especially sweet potatoes, are high in potassium. Consider choosing lower-potassium alternatives like cauliflower, cucumbers, or green beans.

4. Tomatoes and Tomato Products: Tomatoes and tomato-based products like tomato sauce and ketchup are high in potassium. Opt for low-sodium or no-salt-added versions of these products to reduce potassium intake.

5. Dried Fruits: Dried fruits such as raisins, apricots, and prunes are concentrated sources of potassium. Choose fresh fruits instead or limit portion sizes of dried fruits.

6. Avocados: Avocados are a nutrient-dense fruit, but they are also high in potassium. Consider limiting avocado consumption or choosing smaller portions.

7. Spinach and Other Dark Leafy Greens: Dark leafy greens like spinach, kale, and Swiss chard are nutritious but high in potassium. Cook these vegetables to reduce their potassium content or choose lower-potassium alternatives like lettuce or cabbage.

8. Salt Substitutes: Some salt substitutes contain potassium chloride as a replacement for sodium chloride. These should be avoided or used with caution, especially for individuals with kidney disease.

9. Nuts and Seeds: Nuts and seeds are nutritious but can be high in potassium. Consider consuming them in moderation or choosing lower-potassium options like almonds or sunflower seeds.

10. Processed Foods: Processed foods like canned soups, frozen meals, and snack foods often contain added potassium. Check food labels for potassium content and choose low-potassium alternatives.

Chapter 7: Managing Phosphorus Levels

The Importance of Phosphorus Control in Kidney Disease

Phosphorus is a mineral that plays a crucial role in bone health, energy metabolism, and various cellular functions. However, for individuals with kidney disease, especially those with compromised kidney function, maintaining proper phosphorus levels is essential to prevent complications and maintain overall health.

In kidney disease, the kidneys are less effective at filtering and excreting phosphorus from the body. As a result, phosphorus levels can build up in the blood, leading to a condition known as hyperphosphatemia. Elevated phosphorus levels can have several adverse effects, including:

1. Bone Health: High phosphorus levels can disrupt the balance of calcium and phosphorus in the body, leading to weakened bones and an increased risk of fractures.

2. Cardiovascular Health: Elevated phosphorus levels have been associated with an increased risk of cardiovascular disease and mortality in individuals with kidney disease.

3. Mineral and Bone Disorders: Chronic kidney disease-mineral and bone disorder (CKD-MBD) is a common complication of kidney disease characterized by abnormalities in bone and mineral metabolism, including high phosphorus levels.

Managing phosphorus levels in kidney disease involves a combination of dietary changes, medication, and monitoring. Dietary modifications often include:

- Limiting High-Phosphorus Foods: Foods rich in phosphorus, such as dairy products, nuts, seeds, and certain types of meat and fish, may need to be limited or avoided to help control phosphorus intake.

- Phosphate Binders: These medications are often prescribed to help reduce the absorption of phosphorus from the diet, thereby lowering blood phosphorus levels.

- Monitoring Phosphorus Intake: Keeping track of phosphorus intake through food and beverages can help individuals with kidney disease make informed dietary choices and avoid excessive phosphorus consumption.

- Balancing Calcium and Phosphorus Intake: Maintaining a proper balance between calcium and phosphorus intake is important, as these minerals interact closely in the body.

How to limit phosphorus intake while still meeting nutritional needs

- Choose foods with lower phosphorus-to-protein ratios like chicken, beef, eggs and milk. Avoid organ meats like liver which are high in phosphorus.

- Soak high phosphorus foods like beans, grains and nuts to help remove some phosphorus. Rinse canned beans well before cooking.

- Opt for white over whole grain varieties of breads, pastas and cereals. Refining removes some of the phosphorus-rich bran.

- Limit highly processed foods like canned meats, frozen pizza, packaged crackers and cheeses, as additives contain phosphorus.

- Get protein from low phosphorus options like legumes and tofu instead of dairy for some meals.

- Use lemon juice or vinegar to help block phosphorus absorption when cooking vegetables and meats.

- Balance meals with low phosphorus foods like fruits, vegetables, oils and unenriched rice and corn.

- Take a multivitamin to help meet needs for vitamins like calcium and iron that may be limited by restricting dairy and grains.

- Work with a renal dietitian to create a meal plan limiting phosphorus but providing all essential nutrients within individual restrictions.

With careful menu planning, it is possible to restrict phosphorus adequately while maintaining overall nutritional health. Getting regular lab work helps ensure you avoid malnutrition.

Foods high in phosphorus and how to minimize their impact

1. Dairy: Dairy products like cheese, milk, yogurt, and pudding are rich in phosphorus. Opt for lower phosphorus dairy options such as cream, butter, or non-dairy milk substitutes like almond milk or rice milk. These alternatives can provide a similar texture and flavor without the high phosphorus content.

2. Meat and Poultry: Organ meats like liver are very high in phosphorus. Choose lean cuts of beef, pork, chicken, or fish, which generally have lower phosphorus content compared to organ meats.

3. Whole Grains: Whole grains like wheat bran, oatmeal, and brown rice are high in phosphorus. Consider switching to refined grains like white rice or white bread, which typically have lower phosphorus levels. However, it's important to balance this with other dietary considerations, such as fiber intake.

4. Beans and Legumes: Soybeans, lentils, and baked beans are examples of legumes that are high in phosphorus. Opt for legumes with lower phosphorus content, such as green beans or chickpeas. Soaking and rinsing beans before cooking can help reduce their phosphorus content.

5. Nuts and Seeds: Almonds, walnuts, and sunflower seeds are high in phosphorus. Limiting portions of nuts and seeds or avoiding them altogether can help reduce phosphorus intake.

6. Processed Foods: Canned tuna/meats, pre-made baked goods, and frozen pizza often contain added phosphorus. Read labels carefully and avoid products with added phosphoric acid or other phosphorus-containing additives.

7. Beverages: Colas, cocoa, and beer are beverages that can contribute to phosphorus intake. Opt for beverages like coffee, tea, lemonade, or limit the intake of phosphorus-rich drinks.

8. Supplements: Some vitamins or mineral supplements may contain phosphorus additives. Check with your doctor before taking any

supplements to ensure they are appropriate for your dietary needs.

Overall, minimizing meat and dairy portions, limiting processed convenience foods, soaking high phosphorus plant foods, and choosing white over whole grain options can help reduce dietary phosphorus intake. It's important to work with a renal dietitian or healthcare professional to create a personalized meal plan that meets your specific dietary requirements while managing phosphorus levels effectively.

Chapter 8: Fluid Management

The Importance of Fluid Balance in Kidney Disease

Maintaining proper fluid balance is crucial for individuals with compromised kidney function. As kidney disease progresses, the kidneys' ability to filter wastes and extra fluid from the bloodstream becomes impaired. This can lead to fluid overload and electrolyte imbalances if fluid intake is not regulated appropriately.

Excess fluid retention strains the heart and blood vessels, causing swelling, shortness of breath, hypertension, and increased risk of heart failure.

Conversely, removing too much fluid can also be dangerous and lead to dehydration, electrolyte disturbances, and volume depletion. Therefore, meticulous fluid management is a key component of treatment for all stages of chronic kidney disease.

Strict fluid restriction may be recommended, which can be very challenging for patients. Fluid intake from foods, beverages, and intravenous fluids must all be accounted for and added together to stay under the allotted limit. Fluid restriction aims to prevent fluid from accumulating between dialysis sessions for those requiring this treatment.

Here's why fluid management is important in kidney disease:

1. Blood Pressure Regulation: Adequate fluid balance helps regulate blood pressure. In kidney disease, excess fluid retention can lead to high blood pressure (hypertension), which can further damage the kidneys and increase the risk of cardiovascular complications.

2. Electrolyte Balance: Proper fluid balance is essential for maintaining the body's electrolyte levels, including sodium, potassium, and chloride. Electrolyte

imbalances can occur in kidney disease, leading to complications such as muscle cramps, weakness, and irregular heart rhythms.

3. Edema Control: Edema, or swelling due to fluid retention, is a common symptom of kidney disease. Managing fluid intake is crucial for controlling edema and preventing its associated discomfort and complications.

4. Heart Health: Excessive fluid retention can strain the heart, leading to conditions like congestive heart failure. Maintaining a healthy fluid balance is important for supporting heart function, especially in individuals with existing heart or kidney conditions.

5. Dialysis: For individuals on dialysis, managing fluid intake is particularly important, as the dialysis process helps remove excess fluid and waste products from the body. Strict fluid restriction may be necessary for those undergoing dialysis to avoid complications.

Managing fluid intake in kidney disease involves balancing fluid consumption with urine output and other factors such as dietary salt intake and individual health status. This often requires close monitoring of fluid intake and output, as well as working with healthcare providers to develop a personalized fluid management plan.

For individuals in end-stage renal disease, meticulous monitoring of fluid gains and losses is required to guide dialysis prescription. Careful attention must be paid to thirst, blood pressure, edema, and weight changes to achieve optimal fluid status. Ongoing education and support from the healthcare team are essential to help patients understand and comply with prescribed fluid restrictions. Adhering to fluid limits can significantly improve outcomes and quality of life for those living with kidney disease.

Strategies for Managing Fluid Intake and Tips for Thirst Control

1. Fluid Restriction: In some cases of advanced kidney disease, healthcare providers may recommend a fluid restriction to help manage fluid balance. This restriction is individualized based on factors such as urine output, weight changes, and overall health

status. It's important to follow your healthcare provider's guidance regarding fluid intake.

2. Monitoring Fluid Intake: Keeping track of your daily fluid intake can help you stay within your recommended limits. This includes not only beverages but also foods with high water content, such as fruits and vegetables.

3. Thirst Control: Managing thirst can be challenging when on a fluid restriction. Some tips for controlling thirst include rinsing your mouth with cold water, sucking on ice chips, or chewing sugar-free gum or candies to help alleviate dry mouth without consuming excess fluids.

4. Choosing the Right Beverages: When selecting beverages, opt for those that are less likely to contribute to fluid retention. Water is generally the best choice, but other options such as herbal teas, diluted fruit juices, or homemade ice pops made from low-potassium fruits can provide variety while still keeping fluid intake in check.

5. Limiting High-Sodium Foods: Sodium can lead to fluid retention, so it's important to limit high-sodium

foods in your diet. This includes processed foods, canned soups, salty snacks, and fast food. Cooking at home using fresh ingredients and herbs and spices instead of salt can help reduce sodium intake.

6. Incorporating Foods with High Water Content: Foods with high water content, such as cucumbers, lettuce, celery, and watermelon, can contribute to your overall hydration without significantly increasing fluid intake.

7. Working with a Dietitian: A registered dietitian who specializes in kidney health can provide personalized guidance on fluid management, taking into account your individual needs, preferences, and medical history.

Monitoring Signs of Dehydration and Fluid Overload

For individuals with kidney disease, managing fluid intake is essential to maintain proper hydration and prevent complications associated with fluid imbalances. Both dehydration and fluid overload can have serious consequences, so it's crucial to monitor your body's fluid status carefully. Here are some key points to consider:

1. Signs of Dehydration:
   - Thirst: Feeling thirsty is one of the body's first signals of dehydration.
   - Dark Urine: Urine that is dark yellow or amber in color may indicate dehydration.
   - Dry Mouth and Skin: Dryness in the mouth and skin can be signs of inadequate hydration.
   - Fatigue: Dehydration can lead to feelings of fatigue and weakness.
   - Dizziness or Lightheadedness: In some cases, dehydration can cause dizziness or lightheadedness.

2. Signs of Fluid Overload:
   - Swelling (Edema): Fluid buildup in the body can cause swelling, particularly in the legs, ankles, and feet.
   - Shortness of Breath: Excess fluid in the lungs can lead to difficulty breathing or shortness of breath.
   - High Blood Pressure: Fluid overload can contribute to elevated blood pressure.

- Rapid Weight Gain: Sudden weight gain can be a sign of fluid retention.

- Reduced Urination: A decrease in urine output or changes in urine color can indicate fluid retention.

3. Fluid Intake Guidelines:

- Work with your healthcare team to determine your individual fluid intake needs based on your kidney function, overall health, and other factors.

- Monitor your fluid intake by keeping track of the liquids you consume throughout the day.

- Be mindful of your thirst cues and drink water or other fluids when you feel thirsty, but avoid excessive intake.

- Limit fluid intake from sources like soups, ice cream, and fruits with high water content if you are on a fluid-restricted diet.

4. Balancing Fluids:

- Balance your fluid intake with fluid losses, including urine output, sweating, and other factors.

- Be aware of your sodium intake, as sodium can affect fluid balance in the body.

- Discuss any concerns about fluid management with your healthcare team, including changes in your thirst, urine output, or any signs of dehydration or fluid overload.

The optimal fluid intake can vary based on individual factors such as age, gender, body size, activity level, overall health, and kidney function. Here's a general overview of the range of fluid intake based on these factors:

1. Age:
   - Adults: Around 8-10 cups (64-80 ounces) of fluids per day is a common guideline for adults. However, individual needs may vary based on factors like activity level and health status.

2. Gender:
   - Men: Generally have higher fluid needs than women due to differences in body composition and metabolism.
   - Women: May have slightly lower fluid needs compared to men.

3. Body Size:
   - Larger individuals: May require more fluids to maintain hydration compared to smaller individuals.

4. Activity Level:

   - Higher activity levels: Individuals who are more physically active or engage in intense exercise may need more fluids to replace lost fluids through sweat.

5. Overall Health:

   - Certain medical conditions: Some medical conditions may affect fluid needs. For example, individuals with fever, vomiting, or diarrhea may need increased fluids to replace losses.

6. Kidney Function:

   - Individuals with compromised kidney function: Those with kidney disease or on dialysis may need to restrict fluid intake to avoid fluid overload.

It's important to note that these are general guidelines, and individual fluid needs can vary widely. Factors such as climate, altitude, and dietary habits can also influence fluid requirements. For personalized recommendations, it's best to consult with a healthcare provider or registered dietitian who can assess your specific needs and provide tailored guidance.

Chapter 9: Special Considerations for Dialysis Patients

Dietary Recommendations Specific to Individuals Undergoing Dialysis

For individuals undergoing dialysis, dietary considerations play a crucial role in managing their health and well-being. Dialysis is a treatment that helps to remove waste products and excess fluid from the body when the kidneys are no longer able to perform these functions adequately. Here are some dietary recommendations specific to individuals undergoing dialysis:

1. Fluid Intake Management:
   - Dialysis patients often need to restrict their fluid intake to avoid fluid overload, which can lead to complications such as edema and high blood pressure.
   - Monitoring fluid intake carefully and adhering to the prescribed fluid restriction is essential for maintaining a healthy fluid balance.

2. Protein Intake:
   - Protein is important for maintaining muscle mass and overall health, but dialysis patients may need to adjust their protein intake based on their individual needs and the stage of their kidney disease.
   - Working with a dietitian to determine the appropriate amount of protein for their diet can help dialysis patients maintain optimal nutrition without putting excess strain on their kidneys.

3. Phosphorus and Potassium Control:
   - Dialysis patients often need to limit their intake of phosphorus and potassium, as these minerals can

build up in the blood when the kidneys are not functioning properly.

  - Choosing low-phosphorus and low-potassium foods, avoiding high-phosphorus additives, and using phosphate binders as prescribed can help manage these levels.

4. Sodium Restriction:

  - Limiting sodium intake is important for dialysis patients to help control blood pressure and reduce the risk of fluid retention.

  - Avoiding processed and packaged foods, which are often high in sodium, and using herbs and spices to flavor foods instead of salt can help reduce sodium intake.

5. Caloric Needs:

  - Dialysis patients may have different caloric needs based on factors such as age, gender, activity level, and overall health.

  - Working with a dietitian to determine appropriate caloric intake and meal planning can help dialysis patients maintain a healthy weight and meet their nutritional needs.

6. Vitamin and Mineral Supplements:

- Some dialysis patients may require vitamin and mineral supplements, such as vitamin D or iron, to address deficiencies that can occur due to the dialysis process or dietary restrictions.
- It's important to follow the recommendations of a healthcare provider or dietitian regarding supplement use.

7. Individualized Meal Planning:
- Each dialysis patient's dietary needs are unique, and meal planning should be individualized based on their specific health status, nutritional needs, and personal preferences.
- Regular monitoring of nutritional status and adjustments to the meal plan as needed can help dialysis patients maintain optimal health.

The Role of Exercise, Stress Management, and Sleep in Kidney Health

Several lifestyle factors, including regular exercise, effective stress management, and quality sleep, can play a significant role in promoting kidney health. Here's how each of these factors contributes to kidney health:

1. Exercise and Kidney Health:
   - Regular physical activity can help improve cardiovascular health, manage weight, and reduce the risk of chronic diseases such as diabetes and hypertension, which are common risk factors for kidney disease.
   - Exercise can also improve circulation and blood flow, which is important for kidney function.
   - Engaging in regular, moderate-intensity exercise, such as brisk walking, swimming, or cycling, for at least 150 minutes per week is recommended for overall health, including kidney health.

2. Stress Management and Kidney Health:
   - Chronic stress can contribute to the development and progression of kidney disease by affecting blood pressure, immune function, and inflammation.
   - Effective stress management techniques, such as mindfulness meditation, deep breathing exercises, yoga, or engaging in hobbies and activities you enjoy, can help reduce stress levels and promote overall well-being.

3. Sleep and Kidney Health:
   - Quality sleep is essential for overall health, including kidney health. Poor sleep quality or

insufficient sleep can lead to increased inflammation, elevated blood pressure, and impaired immune function, all of which can negatively impact kidney health.

   - Aim for 7-9 hours of quality sleep each night, and practice good sleep hygiene habits, such as maintaining a regular sleep schedule, creating a relaxing bedtime routine, and optimizing your sleep environment.

4. Healthy Lifestyle Choices:
   - In addition to exercise, stress management, and sleep, other lifestyle factors such as maintaining a healthy weight, avoiding smoking and excessive alcohol consumption, and following a balanced diet rich in fruits, vegetables, whole grains, and lean proteins can also support kidney health.
   - Avoiding excessive intake of sodium, phosphorus, and potassium, as well as staying hydrated by drinking an adequate amount of fluids, can also help protect kidney function.

The Role of Exercise, Stress Management, and Sleep in Kidney Health

Maintaining a healthy lifestyle is crucial for supporting kidney health and overall well-being. Several lifestyle factors, including regular exercise, effective stress management, and quality sleep, can play a significant role in promoting kidney health. Here's how each of these factors contributes to kidney health:

1. Exercise and Kidney Health:
  - Regular physical activity can help improve cardiovascular health, manage weight, and reduce the risk of chronic diseases such as diabetes and hypertension, which are common risk factors for kidney disease.
  - Exercise can also improve circulation and blood flow, which is important for kidney function.
  - Engaging in regular, moderate-intensity exercise, such as brisk walking, swimming, or cycling, for at

least 150 minutes per week is recommended for overall health, including kidney health.

2. Stress Management and Kidney Health:
  - Chronic stress can contribute to the development and progression of kidney disease by affecting blood pressure, immune function, and inflammation.
  - Effective stress management techniques, such as mindfulness meditation, deep breathing exercises, yoga, or engaging in hobbies and activities you enjoy, can help reduce stress levels and promote overall well-being.

3. Sleep and Kidney Health:
  - Quality sleep is essential for overall health, including kidney health. Poor sleep quality or insufficient sleep can lead to increased inflammation, elevated blood pressure, and impaired immune function, all of which can negatively impact kidney health.
  - Aim for 7-9 hours of quality sleep each night, and practice good sleep hygiene habits, such as maintaining a regular sleep schedule, creating a relaxing bedtime routine, and optimizing your sleep environment.

4. Healthy Lifestyle Choices:

- In addition to exercise, stress management, and sleep, other lifestyle factors such as maintaining a healthy weight, avoiding smoking and excessive alcohol consumption, and following a balanced diet rich in fruits, vegetables, whole grains, and lean proteins can also support kidney health.

- Avoiding excessive intake of sodium, phosphorus, and potassium, as well as staying hydrated by drinking an adequate amount of fluids, can also help protect kidney function.

Chapter 10: Recipes and Meal Ideas

Kidney-friendly recipes for breakfast, lunch, dinner, and snacks

28-day meal plan for individuals with kidney health considerations. Each day includes breakfast, lunch, dinner, and snacks, along with details on nutrient and energy content.

Week 1

Day 1

Breakfast

- Scrambled Eggs (2 large eggs)
- Whole Grain Toast (1 slice)
- Melon Slices (1 cup)

Lunch

- Turkey Sandwich
  - Whole Wheat Bread (2 slices)
  - Turkey Breast (3 oz.)
  - Lettuce, Tomato, Onion
  - Mustard
- Carrot Sticks (1/2 cup)
- Low-Fat Yogurt (6 oz.)

Dinner

- Baked Salmon (4 oz.)
- Brown Rice (1/2 cup)
- Steamed Broccoli (1 cup)
- Mixed Green Salad with Olive Oil and Lemon Dressing

Snack

- Apple Slices (1 medium)
- Almonds (1/4 cup)

Notes:
- Prepare the scrambled eggs with minimal added salt.

- Choose whole grain bread for the sandwich to increase fiber content.

- Season the salmon with herbs and lemon instead of salt.
- Limit the portion size of almonds to control phosphorus intake.

Nutrient Content:
- Protein: ~75g
- Fiber: ~25g
- Phosphorus: ~700mg
- Sodium: ~1800mg
- Potassium: ~2500mg
- Energy: ~1800 calories

Day 2

Breakfast

- Oatmeal with Berries
  - Steel-Cut Oats (1/2 cup cooked)
  - Mixed Berries (1/2 cup)
  - Almond Milk (unsweetened, 1/2 cup)

Lunch
- Quinoa Salad
  - Quinoa (1/2 cup)
  - Mixed Vegetables (1 cup)
  - Lemon Juice and Olive Oil Dressing

Dinner
- Grilled Chicken Breast (4 oz.)
- Sweet Potato Mash (1/2 cup)
- Steamed Green Beans (1 cup)

Snack
- Greek Yogurt (low-fat, 6 oz.)
- Blueberries (1/2 cup)

Notes:
- Use unsweetened almond milk to reduce added sugars.
- Include a variety of vegetables in the quinoa salad for added nutrients.

- Season the chicken breast with herbs and spices instead of salt.

Nutrient Content:
- Protein: ~70g
- Fiber: ~30g
- Phosphorus: ~600mg
- Sodium: ~1600mg
- Potassium: ~2300mg
- Energy: ~1700 calories

 Day 3

Breakfast
- Whole Grain Waffles (2 pieces)
- Fresh Strawberries (1 cup)
- Maple Syrup (1 tbsp)

Lunch
- Tuna Salad Wrap
  - Whole Wheat Tortilla
  - Tuna Salad (made with low-fat mayo)
  - Lettuce, Tomato
- Orange (1 medium)

Dinner
- Vegetable Stir-Fry with Tofu
  - Tofu (3 oz.)
  - Mixed Vegetables
  - Low-Sodium Soy Sauce
  - Brown Rice (1/2 cup)

Snack
- Cottage Cheese (low-fat, 1/2 cup)
- Pineapple Chunks (1/2 cup)

Notes:
- Choose whole grain waffles for added fiber.
- Use low-sodium soy sauce to reduce sodium intake.
- Limit the portion size of cottage cheese to control phosphorus intake.

Nutrient Content:
- Protein: ~65g
- Fiber: ~20g
- Phosphorus: ~550mg
- Sodium: ~1500mg
- Potassium: ~2200mg
- Energy: ~1600 calories

Day 4

Breakfast
- Greek Yogurt Parfait
  - Greek Yogurt (low-fat, 6 oz.)
  - Granola (1/4 cup)
  - Mixed Berries (1/2 cup)

Lunch
- Chicken Caesar Salad
  - Grilled Chicken Breast (3 oz.)
  - Romaine Lettuce
  - Cherry Tomatoes
  - Parmesan Cheese (1 tbsp)
  - Caesar Dressing (low-sodium)

Dinner
- Lentil Soup
  - Lentils (1/2 cup)
  - Mixed Vegetables
  - Low-Sodium Vegetable Broth

Snack
- Rice Cakes (2 cakes)

- Hummus (2 tbsp)

Notes:
- Choose low-fat Greek yogurt for protein and probiotics.
- Opt for a low-sodium Caesar dressing for the salad.
- Use low-sodium vegetable broth for the lentil soup.

Nutrient Content:
- Protein: ~60g
- Fiber: ~25g
- Phosphorus: ~500mg
- Sodium: ~1400mg
- Potassium: ~2000mg
- Energy: ~1500 calories

Day 5

Breakfast
- Whole Grain Pancakes (2 pieces)
- Banana Slices (1 medium)
- Honey (1 tbsp)

Lunch

- Vegetable and Chickpea Salad
  - Mixed Greens
  - Chickpeas (1/2 cup)
  - Cucumber, Bell Pepper, Red Onion
  - Lemon and Olive Oil Dressing

Dinner
- Grilled Pork Tenderloin (4 oz.)
- Quinoa Pilaf with Vegetables
- Steamed Asparagus (1 cup)

Snack
- Mixed Nuts (1/4 cup)
- Dried Apricots (1/4 cup)

Notes:
- Use whole grain pancake mix for added fiber.
- Include a variety of vegetables in the salad for added nutrients.
- Choose unsalted nuts to limit sodium intake.

Nutrient Content:
- Protein: ~70g
- Fiber: ~30g
- Phosphorus: ~600mg
- Sodium: ~1600mg

- Potassium: ~2300mg
- Energy: ~1700 calories

Day 6

Breakfast
- Scrambled Tofu with Spinach
  - Tofu (4 oz.)
  - Spinach (1 cup)
  - Bell Pepper, Onion
  - Turmeric, Black Pepper
  - Whole Grain Toast (1 slice)

Lunch
- Turkey and Avocado Wrap
  - Whole Wheat Tortilla
  - Turkey Breast (3 oz.)
  - Avocado Slices
  - Lettuce, Tomato
- Carrot Sticks (1/2 cup)
- Low-Fat Yogurt (6 oz.)

Dinner
- Baked Cod (4 oz.)

- Quinoa Salad with Vinaigrette
- Steamed Green Beans (1 cup)

Snack
- Fresh Berries (1/2 cup)
- Cottage Cheese (low-fat, 1/2 cup)

Notes:
- Use tofu as a protein source in the breakfast scramble.
- Include healthy fats from avocado in the wrap.
- Choose a vinaigrette with low sodium content for the quinoa salad.

Nutrient Content:
- Protein: ~65g
- Fiber: ~25g
- Phosphorus: ~550mg
- Sodium: ~1500mg
- Potassium: ~2200mg
- Energy: ~1600 calories

Day 7

Breakfast

- Yogurt and Fruit Parfait
  - Greek Yogurt (low-fat, 6 oz.)
  - Granola (1/4 cup)
  - Mixed Berries (1/2 cup)

Lunch

- Chicken and Vegetable Stir-Fry
  - Chicken Breast (3 oz.)
  - Mixed Vegetables
  - Low-Sodium Soy Sauce
  - Brown Rice (1/2 cup)

Dinner

- Lentil and Vegetable Stew
  - Lentils (1/2 cup)
  - Mixed Vegetables
  - Low-Sodium Vegetable Broth

Snack

- Rice Cakes (2 cakes)
- Hummus (2 tbsp)

Notes:

- Choose low-fat Greek yogurt for the parfait.
- Use low-sodium soy sauce for the stir-fry.

- Prepare the lentil stew with a variety of vegetables for added nutrients.

Nutrient Content:
- Protein: ~60g
- Fiber: ~25g
- Phosphorus: ~500mg
- Sodium: ~1400mg
- Potassium: ~2000mg
- Energy: ~1500 calories

Week 2

Day 8

Breakfast
- Whole Grain Toast with Peanut Butter
- Banana (1 medium)

Lunch
- Tuna Salad
  - Tuna (canned in water, drained)
  - Mixed Greens
  - Cherry Tomatoes

- Low-Fat Salad Dressing

Dinner
- Grilled Chicken Breast (4 oz.)
- Baked Sweet Potato (1 medium)
- Steamed Asparagus (1 cup)

Snack
- Greek Yogurt (low-fat, 6 oz.)
- Blueberries (1/2 cup)

Notes:
- Choose whole grain bread for added fiber in breakfast.
- Use low-fat dressing for the tuna salad.

Nutrient Content:
- Protein: ~70g
- Fiber: ~25g
- Phosphorus: ~600mg
- Sodium: ~1600mg
- Potassium: ~2300mg
- Energy: ~1700 calories

Day 9

Breakfast
- Spinach and Cheese Omelet (2 eggs)
- Whole Grain English Muffin (1 piece)

Lunch
- Turkey and Avocado Wrap
  - Whole Wheat Tortilla
  - Turkey Breast (3 oz.)
  - Avocado Slices
  - Lettuce, Tomato
- Carrot Sticks (1/2 cup)
- Low-Fat Yogurt (6 oz.)

Dinner
- Baked Salmon (4 oz.)
- Quinoa Pilaf with Vegetables
- Steamed Green Beans (1 cup)

Snack
- Fresh Berries (1/2 cup)
- Cottage Cheese (low-fat, 1/2 cup)

Notes:

- Add spinach and low-phosphorus cheese to the
omelet for variety.
- Choose a whole grain English muffin for added fiber.

Nutrient Content:
- Protein: ~65g
- Fiber: ~30g
- Phosphorus: ~600mg
- Sodium: ~1600mg
- Potassium: ~2300mg
- Energy: ~1700 calories

Day 10

Breakfast
- Greek Yogurt with Honey and Almonds
  - Greek Yogurt (low-fat, 6 oz.)
  - Almonds (1/4 cup)
  - Honey (1 tbsp)

Lunch
- Chicken Caesar Salad
  - Grilled Chicken Breast (3 oz.)
  - Romaine Lettuce

  - Cherry Tomatoes
  - Parmesan Cheese (1 tbsp)
  - Caesar Dressing (low-sodium)

Dinner
- Lentil Soup
  - Lentils (1/2 cup)
  - Mixed Vegetables
  - Low-Sodium Vegetable Broth

Snack
- Rice Cakes (2 cakes)
- Hummus (2 tbsp)

Notes:
- Use low-fat Greek yogurt for added protein.
- Opt for a low-sodium Caesar dressing for the salad.
- Use low-sodium vegetable broth for the lentil soup.

Nutrient Content:
- Protein: ~60g
- Fiber: ~25g
- Phosphorus: ~500mg
- Sodium: ~1400mg
- Potassium: ~2000mg
- Energy: ~1500 calories

Day 11

Breakfast
- Whole Grain Pancakes (2 pieces)
- Fresh Berries (1/2 cup)
- Maple Syrup (1 tbsp)

Lunch
- Vegetable and Chickpea Salad
  - Mixed Greens
  - Chickpeas (1/2 cup)
  - Cucumber, Bell Pepper, Red Onion
  - Lemon and Olive Oil Dressing

Dinner
- Grilled Pork Tenderloin (4 oz.)
- Quinoa Salad with Vinaigrette
- Steamed Green Beans (1 cup)

Snack
- Apple Slices (1 medium)
- Almonds (1/4 cup)

Notes:

- Choose whole grain pancake mix for added fiber.
- Include a variety of vegetables in the salad for added nutrients.
- Season the pork tenderloin with herbs and spices instead of salt.

Nutrient Content:
- Protein: ~70g
- Fiber: ~30g
- Phosphorus: ~600mg
- Sodium: ~1600mg
- Potassium: ~2300mg
- Energy: ~1700 calories

Day 12

Breakfast
- Scrambled Tofu with Spinach
  - Tofu (4 oz.)
  - Spinach (1 cup)
  - Bell Pepper, Onion
  - Turmeric, Black Pepper
  - Whole Grain Toast (1 slice)

Lunch
- Turkey and Avocado Wrap
  - Whole Wheat Tortilla
  - Turkey Breast (3 oz.)
  - Avocado Slices
  - Lettuce, Tomato
- Carrot Sticks (1/2 cup)
- Low-Fat Yogurt (6 oz.)

Dinner
- Baked Cod (4 oz.)
- Quinoa Salad with Vinaigrette
- Steamed Green Beans (1 cup)

Snack
- Greek Yogurt (low-fat, 6 oz.)
- Blueberries (1/2 cup)

Notes:
- Use tofu as a protein source in the breakfast scramble.
- Include healthy fats from avocado in the wrap.
- Choose a vinaigrette with low sodium content for the quinoa salad.

Nutrient Content:
- Protein: ~65g
- Fiber: ~25g
- Phosphorus: ~550mg
- Sodium: ~1500mg
- Potassium: ~2200mg
- Energy: ~1600 calories

Day 13

Breakfast
- Yogurt and Fruit Parfait
  - Greek Yogurt (low-fat, 6 oz.)
  - Granola (1/4 cup)
  - Mixed Berries (1/2 cup)

Lunch
- Chicken and Vegetable Stir-Fry
  - Chicken Breast (3 oz.)
  - Mixed Vegetables
  - Low-Sodium Soy Sauce
  - Brown Rice (1/2 cup)

Dinner

- Lentil and Vegetable Stew
  - Lentils (1/2 cup)
  - Mixed Vegetables
  - Low-Sodium Vegetable Broth

Snack
- Rice Cakes (2 cakes)
- Hummus (2 tbsp)

Notes:
- Choose low-fat Greek yogurt for the parfait.
- Use low-sodium soy sauce for the stir-fry.
- Prepare the lentil stew with a variety of vegetables
for added nutrients.

Nutrient Content:
- Protein: ~60g
- Fiber: ~25g
- Phosphorus: ~500mg
- Sodium: ~1400mg
- Potassium: ~2000mg
- Energy: ~1500 calories

Day 14

Breakfast
- Spinach and Cheese Omelet (2 eggs)
- Whole Grain English Muffin (1 piece)

Lunch
- Turkey and Avocado Wrap
  - Whole Wheat Tortilla
  - Turkey Breast (3 oz.)
  - Avocado Slices
  - Lettuce, Tomato
- Carrot Sticks (1/2 cup)
- Low-Fat Yogurt (6 oz.)

Dinner
- Baked Salmon (4 oz.)
- Quinoa Pilaf with Vegetables
- Steamed Green Beans (1 cup)

Snack
- Fresh Berries (1/2 cup)
- Cottage Cheese (low-fat, 1/2 cup)

Notes:
- Add spinach and low-phosphorus cheese to the omelet for variety.

- Choose a whole grain English muffin for added fiber.

Nutrient Content:
- Protein: ~65g
- Fiber: ~30g
- Phosphorus: ~600mg
- Sodium: ~1600mg
- Potassium: ~2300mg
- Energy: ~1700 calories

Week 3

Day 15

Breakfast
- Whole Grain Pancakes (2 pieces)
- Fresh Berries (1/2 cup)
- Maple Syrup (1 tbsp)

Lunch
- Vegetable and Chickpea Salad
  - Mixed Greens
  - Chickpeas (1/2 cup)
  - Cucumber, Bell Pepper, Red Onion

  - Lemon and Olive Oil Dressing

Dinner
- Grilled Pork Tenderloin (4 oz.)
- Quinoa Salad with Vinaigrette
- Steamed Green Beans (1 cup)

Snack
- Apple Slices (1 medium)
- Almonds (1/4 cup)

Notes:
- Choose whole grain pancake mix for added fiber.
- Include a variety of vegetables in the salad for added nutrients.
- Season the pork tenderloin with herbs and spices instead of salt.

Nutrient Content:
- Protein: ~70g
- Fiber: ~30g
- Phosphorus: ~600mg
- Sodium: ~1600mg
- Potassium: ~2300mg
- Energy: ~1700 calories

Day 16

Breakfast
- Greek Yogurt with Honey and Almonds
  - Greek Yogurt (low-fat, 6 oz.)
  - Almonds (1/4 cup)
  - Honey (1 tbsp)

Lunch
- Chicken Caesar Salad
  - Grilled Chicken Breast (3 oz.)
  - Romaine Lettuce
  - Cherry Tomatoes
  - Parmesan Cheese (1 tbsp)
  - Caesar Dressing (low-sodium)

Dinner
- Lentil Soup
  - Lentils (1/2 cup)
  - Mixed Vegetables
  - Low-Sodium Vegetable Broth

Snack
- Rice Cakes (2 cakes)

- Hummus (2 tbsp)

Notes:
- Use low-fat Greek yogurt for added protein.
- Opt for a low-sodium Caesar dressing for the salad.
- Use low-sodium vegetable broth for the lentil soup.

Nutrient Content:
- Protein: ~60g
- Fiber: ~25g
- Phosphorus: ~500mg
- Sodium: ~1400mg
- Potassium: ~2000mg
- Energy: ~1500 calories

Day 17

Breakfast
- Whole Grain Pancakes (2 pieces)
- Fresh Berries (1/2 cup)
- Maple Syrup (1 tbsp)

Lunch
- Turkey and Avocado Wrap

  - Whole Wheat Tortilla
  - Turkey Breast (3 oz.)
  - Avocado Slices
  - Lettuce, Tomato
- Carrot Sticks (1/2 cup)
- Low-Fat Yogurt (6 oz.)

Dinner
- Baked Salmon (4 oz.)
- Quinoa Pilaf with Vegetables
- Steamed Green Beans (1 cup)

Snack
- Fresh Berries (1/2 cup)
- Cottage Cheese (low-fat, 1/2 cup)

Notes:
- Choose whole grain pancake mix for added fiber.
- Include a variety of vegetables in the salad for added nutrients.
- Season the salmon with herbs and spices instead of salt.

Nutrient Content:
- Protein: ~65g
- Fiber: ~30g

- Phosphorus: ~600mg
- Sodium: ~1600mg
- Potassium: ~2300mg
- Energy: ~1700 calories

 Day 18

Breakfast
- Greek Yogurt with Honey and Almonds
  - Greek Yogurt (low-fat, 6 oz.)
  - Almonds (1/4 cup)
  - Honey (1 tbsp)

Lunch
- Chicken and Vegetable Stir-Fry
  - Chicken Breast (3 oz.)
  - Mixed Vegetables
  - Low-Sodium Soy Sauce
  - Brown Rice (1/2 cup)

Dinner
- Lentil and Vegetable Stew
  - Lentils (1/2 cup)
  - Mixed Vegetables

  - Low-Sodium Vegetable Broth

Snack
- Rice Cakes (2 cakes)
- Hummus (2 tbsp)

Notes:
- Use low-fat Greek yogurt for added protein.
- Opt for a low-sodium soy sauce for the stir-fry.
- Use low-sodium vegetable broth for the lentil stew.

Nutrient Content:
- Protein: ~60g
- Fiber: ~25g
- Phosphorus: ~500mg
- Sodium: ~1400mg
- Potassium: ~2000mg
- Energy: ~1500 calories

Day 19

Breakfast
- Spinach and Cheese Omelet (2 eggs)
- Whole Grain English Muffin (1 piece)

Lunch
- Turkey and Avocado Wrap
  - Whole Wheat Tortilla
  - Turkey Breast (3 oz.)
  - Avocado Slices
  - Lettuce, Tomato
- Carrot Sticks (1/2 cup)
- Low-Fat Yogurt (6 oz.)

Dinner
- Baked Salmon (4 oz.)
- Quinoa Pilaf with Vegetables
- Steamed Green Beans (1 cup)

Snack
- Fresh Berries (1/2 cup)
- Cottage Cheese (low-fat, 1/2 cup)

Notes:
- Add spinach and low-phosphorus cheese to the omelet for variety.
- Choose a whole grain English muffin for added fiber.

Nutrient Content:
- Protein: ~65g

- Fiber: ~30g

- Phosphorus: ~600mg

- Sodium: ~1600mg

- Potassium: ~2300mg

- Energy: ~1700 calories

Day 20

Breakfast
- Greek Yogurt with Honey and Almonds
  - Greek Yogurt (low-fat, 6 oz.)
  - Almonds (1/4 cup)
  - Honey (1 tbsp)

Lunch
- Chicken Caesar Salad
  - Grilled Chicken Breast (3 oz.)
  - Romaine Lettuce
  - Cherry Tomatoes
  - Parmesan Cheese (1 tbsp)
  - Caesar Dressing (low-sodium)

Dinner
- Lentil Soup

- Lentils (1/2 cup)
- Mixed Vegetables
- Low-Sodium Vegetable Broth

Snack
- Rice Cakes (2 cakes)
- Hummus (2 tbsp)

Notes:
- Use low-fat Greek yogurt for added protein.
- Opt for a low-sodium Caesar dressing for the salad.
- Use low-sodium vegetable broth for the lentil soup.

Nutrient Content:
- Protein: ~60g
- Fiber: ~25g
- Phosphorus: ~500mg
- Sodium: ~1400mg
- Potassium: ~2000mg
- Energy: ~1500 calories

Day 21

Breakfast

- Whole Grain Pancakes (2 pieces)
- Fresh Berries (1/2 cup)
- Maple Syrup (1 tbsp)

Lunch
- Turkey and Avocado Wrap
  - Whole Wheat Tortilla
  - Turkey Breast (3 oz.)
  - Avocado Slices
  - Lettuce, Tomato
- Carrot Sticks (1/2 cup)
- Low-Fat Yogurt (6 oz.)

Dinner
- Baked Salmon (4 oz.)
- Quinoa Pilaf with Vegetables
- Steamed Green Beans (1 cup)

Snack
- Fresh Berries (1/2 cup)
- Cottage Cheese (low-fat, 1/2 cup)

Notes:
- Choose whole grain pancake mix for added fiber.
- Include a variety of vegetables in the salad for added nutrients.

- Season the salmon with herbs and spices instead of salt.

Nutrient Content:
- Protein: ~65g
- Fiber: ~30g
- Phosphorus: ~600mg
- Sodium: ~1600mg
- Potassium: ~2300mg
- Energy: ~1700 calories

Day 22

Breakfast
- Scrambled Eggs with Spinach and Feta
- Whole Wheat Toast (1 slice)

Lunch
- Tuna Salad Sandwich
  - Whole Grain Bread
  - Tuna Salad with Low-Fat Mayo
  - Lettuce, Tomato
- Carrot Sticks (1/2 cup)
- Low-Fat Yogurt (6 oz.)

Dinner
- Grilled Chicken Breast (4 oz.)
- Quinoa Pilaf with Vegetables
- Steamed Asparagus (1 cup)

Snack
- Apple Slices (1 medium)
- Almonds (1/4 cup)

Notes:
- Use low-fat feta cheese for less sodium.
- Season the chicken breast with herbs and spices instead of salt.

Nutrient Content:
- Protein: ~70g
- Fiber: ~30g
- Phosphorus: ~600mg
- Sodium: ~1600mg
- Potassium: ~2300mg
- Energy: ~1700 calories

Day 23

Breakfast
- Greek Yogurt with Honey and Almonds
  - Greek Yogurt (low-fat, 6 oz.)
  - Almonds (1/4 cup)
  - Honey (1 tbsp)

Lunch
- Chicken and Vegetable Stir-Fry
  - Chicken Breast (3 oz.)
  - Mixed Vegetables
  - Low-Sodium Soy Sauce
  - Brown Rice (1/2 cup)

Dinner
- Lentil and Vegetable Stew
  - Lentils (1/2 cup)
  - Mixed Vegetables
  - Low-Sodium Vegetable Broth

Snack
- Rice Cakes (2 cakes)
- Hummus (2 tbsp)

Notes:
- Use low-fat Greek yogurt for added protein.

- Opt for a low-sodium soy sauce for the stir-fry.
- Use low-sodium vegetable broth for the lentil stew.

Nutrient Content:
- Protein: ~60g
- Fiber: ~25g
- Phosphorus: ~500mg
- Sodium: ~1400mg
- Potassium: ~2000mg
- Energy: ~1500 calories

Day 24

Breakfast
- Spinach and Cheese Omelet (2 eggs)
- Whole Grain English Muffin (1 piece)

Lunch
- Turkey and Avocado Wrap
  - Whole Wheat Tortilla
  - Turkey Breast (3 oz.)
  - Avocado Slices
  - Lettuce, Tomato
- Carrot Sticks (1/2 cup)

- Low-Fat Yogurt (6 oz.)

Dinner
- Baked Salmon (4 oz.)
- Quinoa Pilaf with Vegetables
- Steamed Green Beans (1 cup)

Snack
- Fresh Berries (1/2 cup)
- Cottage Cheese (low-fat, 1/2 cup)

Notes:
- Add spinach and low-phosphorus cheese to the omelet for variety.
- Choose a whole grain English muffin for added fiber.

Nutrient Content:
- Protein: ~65g
- Fiber: ~30g
- Phosphorus: ~600mg
- Sodium: ~1600mg
- Potassium: ~2300mg
- Energy: ~1700 calories

Day 25

Breakfast
- Greek Yogurt with Honey and Almonds
  - Greek Yogurt (low-fat, 6 oz.)
  - Almonds (1/4 cup)
  - Honey (1 tbsp)

Lunch
- Chicken Caesar Salad
  - Grilled Chicken Breast (3 oz.)
  - Romaine Lettuce
  - Cherry Tomatoes
  - Parmesan Cheese (1 tbsp)
  - Caesar Dressing (low-sodium)

Dinner
- Lentil Soup
  - Lentils (1/2 cup)
  - Mixed Vegetables
  - Low-Sodium Vegetable Broth

Snack
- Rice Cakes (2 cakes)
- Hummus (2 tbsp)

Notes:
- Use low-fat Greek yogurt for added protein.
- Opt for a low-sodium Caesar dressing for the salad.
- Use low-sodium vegetable broth for the lentil soup.

Nutrient Content:
- Protein: ~60g
- Fiber: ~25g
- Phosphorus: ~500mg
- Sodium: ~1400mg
- Potassium: ~2000mg
- Energy: ~1500 calories

Day 26

Breakfast
- Whole Grain Pancakes (2 pieces)
- Fresh Berries (1/2 cup)
- Maple Syrup (1 tbsp)

Lunch
- Turkey and Avocado Wrap
  - Whole Wheat Tortilla
  - Turkey Breast (3 oz.)

- Avocado Slices
- Lettuce, Tomato
- Carrot Sticks (1/2 cup)
- Low-Fat Yogurt (6 oz.)

Dinner
- Baked Salmon (4 oz.)
- Quinoa Pilaf with Vegetables
- Steamed Green Beans (1 cup)

Snack
- Fresh Berries (1/2 cup)
- Cottage Cheese (low-fat, 1/2 cup)

Notes:
- Choose whole grain pancake mix for added fiber.
- Include a variety of vegetables in the salad for added nutrients.
- Season the salmon with herbs and spices instead of salt.

Nutrient Content:
- Protein: ~65g
- Fiber: ~30g
- Phosphorus: ~600mg
- Sodium: ~1600mg

- Potassium: ~2300mg
- Energy: ~1700 calories

Day 27

Breakfast
- Greek Yogurt with Honey and Almonds
  - Greek Yogurt (low-fat, 6 oz.)
  - Almonds (1/4 cup)
  - Honey (1 tbsp)

Lunch
- Chicken and Vegetable Stir-Fry
  - Chicken Breast (3 oz.)
  - Mixed Vegetables
  - Low-Sodium Soy Sauce
  - Brown Rice (1/2 cup)

Dinner
- Lentil and Vegetable Stew
  - Lentils (1/2 cup)
  - Mixed Vegetables
  - Low-Sodium Vegetable Broth

Snack

- Rice Cakes (2 cakes)
- Hummus (2 tbsp)

Notes:

- Use low-fat Greek yogurt for added protein.
- Opt for a low-sodium soy sauce for the stir-fry.
- Use low-sodium vegetable broth for the lentil stew.

Nutrient Content:

- Protein: ~60g
- Fiber: ~25g
- Phosphorus: ~500mg
- Sodium: ~1400mg
- Potassium: ~2000mg
- Energy: ~1500 calories

Day 28

Breakfast

- Spinach and Cheese Omelet (2 eggs)
- Whole Grain English Muffin (1 piece)

Lunch

- Turkey and Avocado Wrap
  - Whole Wheat Tortilla
  - Turkey Breast (3 oz.)
  - Avocado Slices
  - Lettuce, Tomato
- Carrot Sticks (1/2 cup)
- Low-Fat Yogurt (6 oz.)

Dinner

- Baked Salmon (4 oz.)
- Quinoa Pilaf with Vegetables
- Steamed Green Beans (1 cup)

Snack

- Fresh Berries (1/2 cup)
- Cottage Cheese (low-fat, 1/2 cup)

Notes:

- Add spinach and low-phosphorus cheese to the omelet for variety.
- Choose a whole grain English muffin for added fiber.

Nutrient Content:

- Protein: ~65g
- Fiber: ~30g
- Phosphorus: ~600mg

- Sodium: ~1600mg
- Potassium: ~2300mg
- Energy: ~1700 calories

This meal plan provides a variety of nutrient-dense foods while paying attention to protein, fiber, phosphorus, sodium, potassium, and overall calorie intake. It is essential to personalize this plan according to individual dietary needs, preferences, and any specific recommendations from a healthcare provider or dietitian.